I0415234

ENDORSEMENTS

"I am a 67-year-old male, and have had hearing loss for over 60 years. Had this book been available, it would have saved my wife and me 34 years of unanswered questions and frustrations. *The Five Keys To Communication Success* is an imperative read for anyone considering hearing aids and those who are early in their hearing aid experience."

Kenneth John Walsh
Retired Christian Schools Superintendent

"The information in this book reinforces communication tools that we, as audiologists, strive to provide our patients throughout the entire evaluation and rehabilitative process. I am excited to provide this book to my patients and their family members. It will help facilitate awareness, knowledge, and realistic expectations about hearing loss for all parties involved, which will then lead to a more effective communication process. Thank you for your amazing contribution to our profession."

Jayme L. Rinn, M.A., CCC-A
Audiologist, Owner of Arvada Hearing Center, Inc.

"As an ENT doctor, I feel Dr. Dusty Jessen's book is a wonderful addition to the world of listening, hearing, and communicating. Dr. Jessen's book will help people to maximize these skills as they enter the world of hearing aids. I also love the clever little dog and bright colors. It was an easy and informative read."

Janice L. Birney, M.D.
Owner, Janice L. Birney, M.D., P.C.

"My husband and I have been married for 34 years, and he has had hearing loss since he was a child. This book taught me things that I never knew. It is equally important for the spouse to understand the *The Five Keys To Communication Success* to help ensure a better quality of life for both partners. I highly recommend this book."

Dr. Pamela Day Walsh

"At last, a book that truly tells it like it is. Too often consumer books and self-help books written by professionals extol the virtues of modern technology while minimizing the adverse effects of human behavior. While it is true that modern technology has progressed significantly, good communication requires more than simply placing hearing aids on your ears. In this easy-to-read guide to better communication, Dr. Jessen places responsibility right where it belongs; on both the listener and those who communicate with the listener, without assigning blame or 'sugar-coating' the situation. She carefully contrasts hearing loss from communication breakdowns and offers constructive, realistic solutions discussed in an environment-specific format. If the reader combines new technology with the words of experienced wisdom contained in this book, optimizing communication despite having a hearing loss can actually be achieved."

Robert W. Sweetow, Ph.D.
Professor of Otolaryngology and Audiology
University of California, San Francisco

Frustrated by Hearing Loss?

5 Keys to
Communication Success

Dusty Ann Jessen, Au.D.

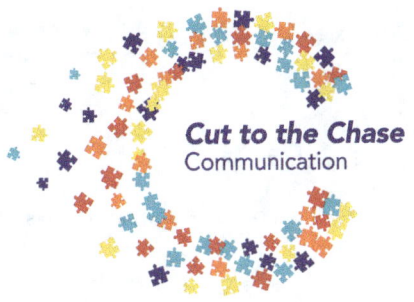

Cut to the Chase
Communication

Frustrated by Hearing Loss?
5 Keys to Communication Success

©2013, 2020 Cut to the Chase Communication, LLC

All rights reserved. This book, or parts thereof, may not be used or reproduced in any form without permission by Cut to the Chase Communication, LLC.

Book Design by Ideas By Nature and Image Resource

First Edition
ISBN 978-1-4675-8104-2 (spiral-bound)
ISBN 978-1-0922-4996-6 (perfect-bound)

To contact the author or for bulk orders: support@5keys.org

www.5keys.info

This book is dedicated to my wonderful patients who give me daily insight into the frustrations, adaptations, and finally the celebrations that occur when practicing the Five Keys to Communication Success.

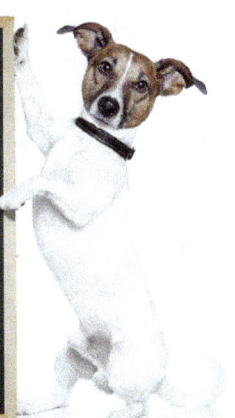

ACKNOWLEDGMENTS

I'd like to thank my colleagues who have dedicated
their lives to helping people with hearing loss.
You are much more than hearing care providers.
You give the gift of communication, self-confidence,
and strengthened relationships to those you serve.

CONTENTS

Section 1

Section 2

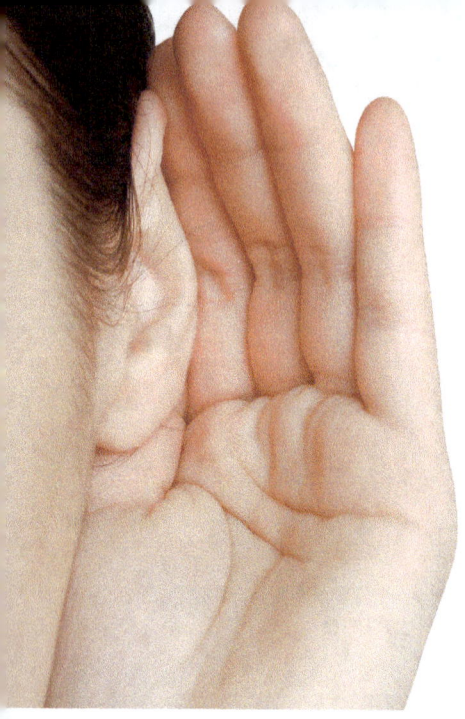

INTRODUCTION

If you find yourself reading this now, chances are that you or someone in your life suffers from hearing loss. Hearing loss is an invisible disability that can cause incredible frustration between family members, friends, and colleagues. It can wreak havoc in the home, in the car, at work, in restaurants, and in many other social situations. In most cases, people lose their hearing gradually, so the signs and symptoms are hard to detect in the beginning. It may begin with a gradual boost of the TV volume, or a mild struggle to catch all parts of a conversation in a noisy restaurant. As hearing loss progresses, people find themselves avoiding certain social situations, struggling to communicate in the workplace or on the phone, and withdrawing from the world in general. What may be surprising is that the detrimental effects of hearing loss are often more disturbing to family, friends, and co-workers than they are to the person with hearing loss. Why is this?

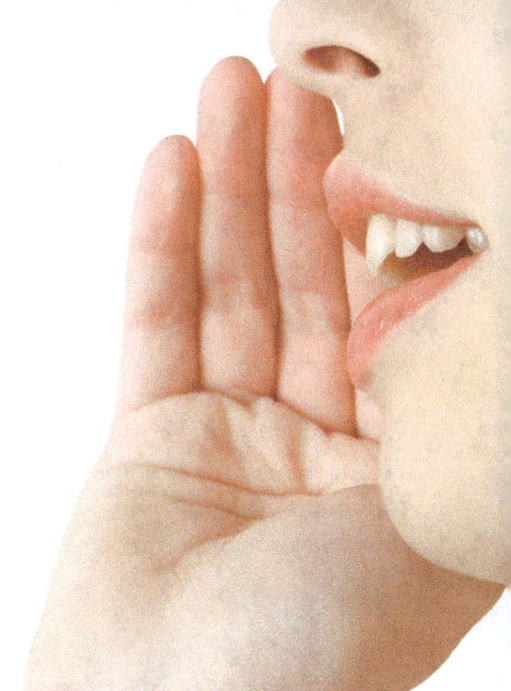

A no-nonsense guide to help you conquer communication breakdowns caused by hearing loss.

Check out this very common scenario:

Meet Mr. and Mrs. Jones. Mr. Jones has slowly lost his hearing over the past several years and finds himself saying "What?" more and more often. His wife is tired of repeating herself and sick of trying to talk over the blaring TV. This loving couple finds themselves increasingly frustrated with each other, all because of...Mr. Jones's hearing loss, right? WRONG!

The frustration is caused by a breakdown in communication. Now don't get me wrong, hearing loss is frustrating for all parties involved. However, there are always at least TWO people involved in any communication exchange, and thus in any communication breakdown. The goal of this handbook is to arm BOTH parties with common sense tools that will make communication easier and more enjoyable in all areas of life.

**Get ready to learn the
Five Keys to Communication Success:**

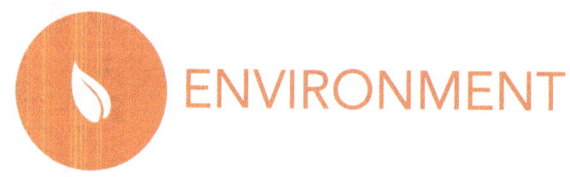

ENVIRONMENT

It is much easier to communicate in a calm and quiet environment. Both the speaker and the listener are responsible for modifying their surroundings to ensure a successful communication exchange.

SPEAKER

If a speaker truly wants to get a message across to the listener, he or she must use effective speaking strategies. It is the speaker's responsibility to learn these strategies and use them in every situation.

LISTENER

There is a big difference between hearing and listening. The listener must learn and use effective listening strategies to receive a message successfully. These strategies apply to listeners with normal hearing as well as those with hearing loss.

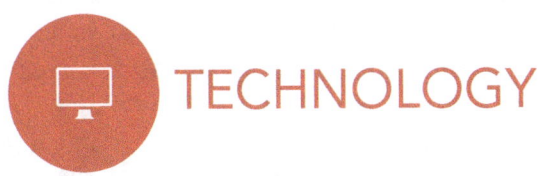

TECHNOLOGY

There are many technological options for people who are experiencing communication breakdowns. Hearing aids, cochlear implants, and assistive listening devices will help significantly when they are programmed and used appropriately.

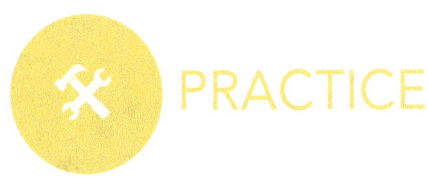

PRACTICE

New habits are not formed overnight. Most people have developed bad communication habits over many years. The keys listed above and described in this handbook will only result in successful communication when they are practiced in every situation.

The following pages will help you to apply these five techniques in several different situations that are notorious for creating communication challenges. After each environment, there is a Successful Communication Plan worksheet to help identify where and with whom the communication breakdown is occurring. The plan will provide guidance for both the speaker and the listener as they apply the keys and create good communication habits. Simply cut out the completed plans from the handbook and post them where they will serve as a constant reminder to practice the following strategies. You can download additional blank Communication Plans from www.5keys.info.

IT TAKES TWO TO TANGO

The following information, when put to use by BOTH communication partners, has the very powerful ability to save relationships, save jobs, and save sanity! It cannot be stressed enough that both parties must read this handbook, and both parties must implement the communication tips. It simply does not work for Mr. Jones to go home and tell Mrs. Jones, "The audiologist says you need to look at me when you speak." In fact, this has the potential to cause more trouble than the communication breakdown itself. It is imperative that the person with hearing loss and ANYONE who wishes to communicate more effectively with that person read this handbook personally.

This handbook is less about hearing loss, and more about COMMUNICATION. The *American Heritage College Dictionary* defines communication as:

- The exchange of thoughts, messages, or information.

- Interpersonal rapport.

- The art and technique of using words effectively in imparting one's ideas.

The second definition really stands out. "Interpersonal rapport" is another way of saying *quality relationships*. Most hearing care providers have been through countless appointments with patients and their spouses discussing this very topic. These sessions can be very emotional and slightly uncomfortable. At times it may feel more like marriage counseling than hearing care, but when both partners implement the following strategies, their interpersonal rapport improves and their relationship strengthens.

The key word in the third definition of communication is "effectively." Communication simply will not occur if the words are not effective in getting the meaning across. If Mr. Jones hears "I need a loaf of bread" when Mrs. Jones tells him "I need to go to bed" then those words were not used effectively and a communication breakdown has occurred.

The workplace is often a difficult situation for people with hearing loss, so it is critical to share this information with co-workers. Meetings and conference calls present unique challenges, as participants are often distracted by their phones or computers and do not put the necessary effort into communicating clearly. In today's fast-paced and technology-driven world, we all need to take a step back and remember to practice the simple yet effective communication strategies discussed throughout this handbook.

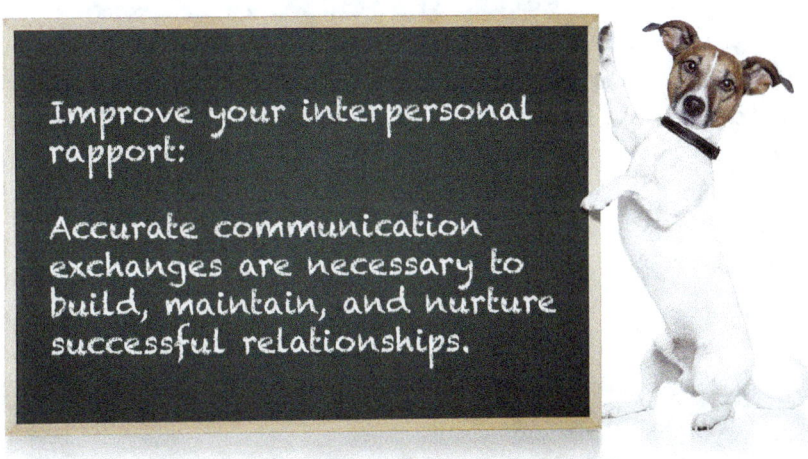

Improve your interpersonal rapport:

Accurate communication exchanges are necessary to build, maintain, and nurture successful relationships.

Note: For the sake of simplicity, we refer to hearing aids throughout this handbook. However, the helpful expectations and technology tips provided in the following pages are just as applicable to those with cochlear implants and other hearing devices.

I JUST SPENT THOUSANDS OF DOLLARS ON NEW HEARING AIDS... DO I NEED TO KEEP READING?

Absolutely! First, congratulations on your commitment to improving your communication with new hearing aids. Today's hearing aids provide better quality hearing than ever before. Technology has come a long way in recent years, and the more advanced hearing aids now allow people with hearing loss to return to activities they may have previously avoided.

Hearing aids can help you reclaim much of the speech and other sounds you have been missing. However, even the most advanced hearing aids will not restore your hearing to normal.

The key to realizing the wonderful benefits of hearing aids is to keep your expectations realistic and know that they are only one piece of the puzzle.

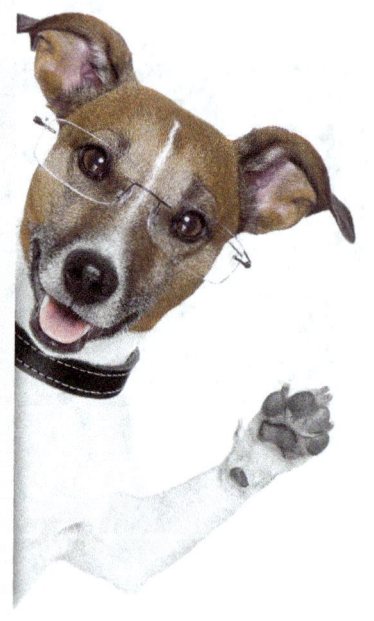

Hearing aids will do their part, but much of the success you receive from them must come from you and the people speaking to you.

Hearing aids will do their part, but much of the success you receive from them must come from you and the people speaking to you.

Many people mistakenly believe that hearing aids only amplify speech and nothing else. However, there are many environmental sounds you need to be able to hear for your enjoyment as well as safety. If hearing aids only amplified speech, you would not hear your telephone ring, birds singing, your smoke alarm, or a car coming down the street. Today's circuitry can analyze speech differently from noise. It can help you hear through noise, but it is not possible nor desirable to eliminate all background noises. When all of these sounds are suddenly restored with your hearing aids, your brain, which may have "forgotten" many sounds, will at first be distracted by each new sound you hear. It takes time to become re-accustomed to the world of sound.

When you first start to wear your hearing aids, the world around you may seem very noisy. In addition to the soft sounds of speech you have been missing, many other sounds will reappear such as paper shuffling, leaves rustling, water dripping, and your microwave running. These are sounds you may not have heard for several years. Over time, as your brain learns to identify important from unimportant sounds, they will become less distracting.

If you wear your aids only occasionally, your brain will never get accustomed to hearing with hearing aids, and they will likely end up in your dresser drawer. Remember, people with normal hearing can hear all of the background noise too, but they have learned to push it out of conscious awareness. You will relearn to do this as well with continual and regular use of your hearing aids.

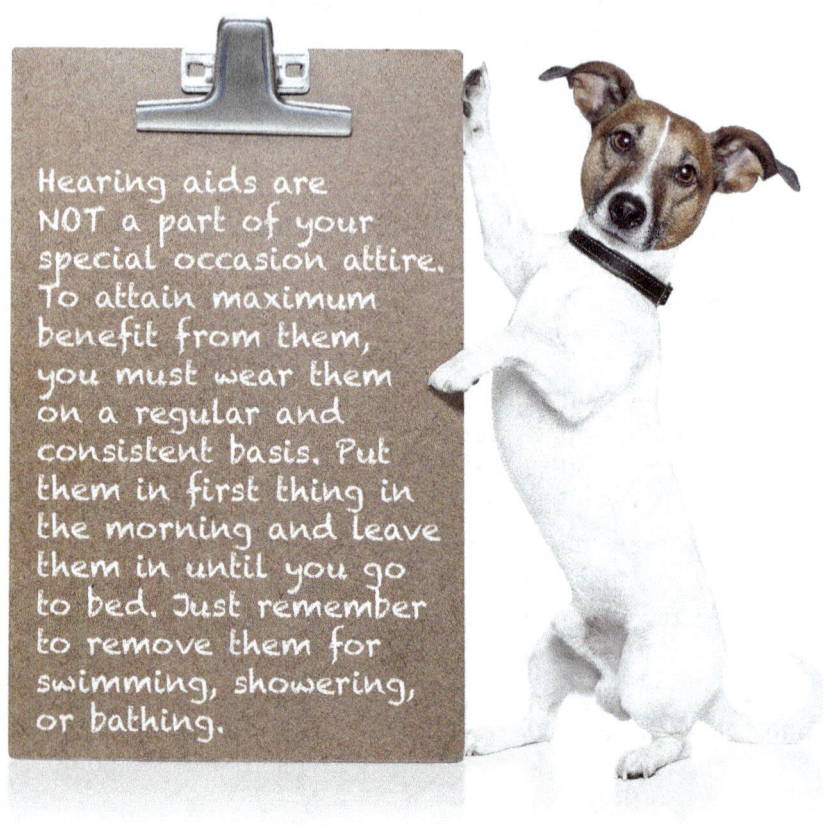

Hearing aids are NOT a part of your special occasion attire. To attain maximum benefit from them, you must wear them on a regular and consistent basis. Put them in first thing in the morning and leave them in until you go to bed. Just remember to remove them for swimming, showering, or bathing.

Some people have trouble understanding speech clearly even when it is made loud enough. Hearing care providers call this "poor word recognition" and will test for it during your initial evaluation. Poor word recognition is common, especially as we get older and our processing abilities begin to slow down a bit. Those with poor word recognition scores can still benefit from hearing aids. However, it is important to know that hearing aids cannot address this challenge alone. It is critical for those with poor word recognition to implement the strategies in this handbook. There are also special auditory training programs designed to improve speech understanding. Ask your hearing care provider if this additional training might be helpful for you.

Helpful Hearing Aid Expectations

- Hearing aids are only one piece of the communication puzzle.

- It will take time to adjust to hearing aids and to realize their full potential.

- Some sounds may be strange initially, including your voice, footsteps, birds, and newspapers.

- Hearing in quiet and mild to moderate background noise should be improved, but hearing in noise will not be as good as hearing in quiet.

- Soft speech should be audible, conversational speech comfortable, and loud speech not uncomfortable.

- No whistling should occur if the hearing aids are seated properly.

- Your own voice may sound different when you are wearing hearing aids.

- Talking on the phone may feel awkward at first as you experiment with proper phone placement and different technology options.

- It is absolutely necessary to return to your hearing care provider for follow up visits and fine-tuning adjustments to the hearing aids.

- Treat yourself to easy listening situations (one-on-one conversations in quiet environments) during the first few days or weeks with the hearing aids as your brain adjusts to hearing again.

- You will benefit most from hearing aids if you use the strategies in this handbook and share them with everyone who communicates with you.

NO-NONSENSE AND COMMON SENSE

It is amazing how often hearing aids are fit on patients, and immediately their family members will go to the opposite side of the office, turn their backs toward the patient, and WHISPER a question. WHAT??? If hearing care providers with normal hearing cannot hear what is whispered, how in the world is the person with hearing loss supposed to hear it? Hearing aids do not give people "super human" hearing, but often this is what is expected of them.

This handbook is going to squash any unrealistic expectations. We are talking about no-nonsense and common sense communication. Interestingly, common sense often flies out the door when we are communicating with people we love.

Let us return to Mr. and Mrs. Jones. Remember, Mr. Jones has a hearing loss, and is really struggling to hear Mrs. Jones around the house. However, when Mrs. Jones is talking to a friend on the telephone, he can hear every word she says, even when he is in another room. Why is this?

This is actually quite common. Mrs. Jones puts more effort into speaking clearly and loudly for her friend to hear. She really wants to get her message across to her friend (building that "interpersonal rapport" or nurturing that friendship) and therefore she does what is needed to achieve that goal. This is wonderful, effective communication on Mrs. Jones' part. However, when she hangs up the phone and starts telling Mr. Jones about her conversation, she drops her volume and talks faster. It also does not help that Mr. Jones is on the other side of the room, next to a TV with the volume blaring so he can hear it.

Sound familiar? Common sense tells us that Mr. Jones will not understand what Mrs. Jones is telling him, but this scenario is repeated multiple times a day in thousands of households around the world.

We tend to communicate least effectively with those we spend time with the most. We get into years and years of bad habits. We get lazy. We each expect the other person to fix the problem. It happens over and over again with very loving (yet frustrated) relationships. Let's change that!

· ·

"My husband and I have been married for 34 years, and he has had hearing loss since he was a child. This book taught me things that I never knew. It is equally important for the spouse to understand the Five Keys to Communication Success to help ensure a better quality of life for both partners."
— PAMELA W.

EFFECTIVE COMMUNICATION BY ENVIRONMENT

It is most often the environment, or situation, that dictates the communication difficulty. Therefore, the remainder of this handbook is divided into different environments to make it a quick-and-easy reference guide for you. If you find yourself in a situation where you are experiencing a communication breakdown, you can quickly flip to that particular environment in this handbook. For example, if you are dining out with your family tonight, you can quickly review the "Dining Out" chapter, and within a couple of minutes you will have environmental, speaker, listener, and technology tips at your fingertips. You will be ready to conquer those potential communication breakdowns that commonly happen in noisy restaurants, and enjoy a pleasant evening with your family.

Obviously it will be more useful for you to read about that particular situation ahead of time so that you can make the necessary preparations, but there will always be tips that you can use in a last-minute communication emergency. This information will equip and empower you to have an effective communication exchange and nurture your most important relationships.

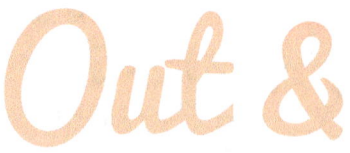

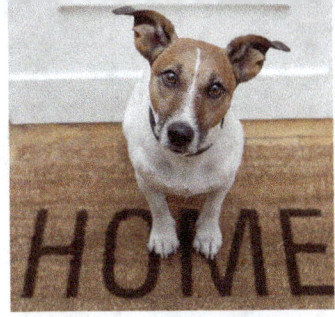

The following environments will be addressed:

- Around the House

- In the Car

- Dining Out

- On the Phone

- Public Events:
  Churches
  Concerts
  Plays
  Large Meetings

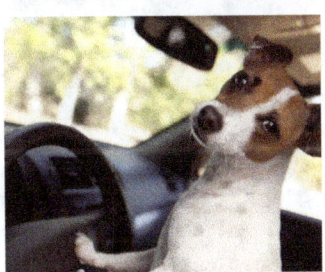

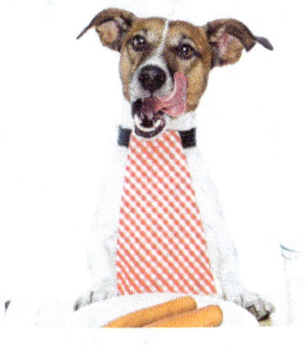

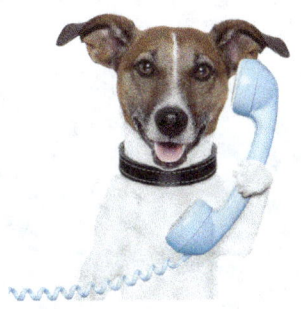

About

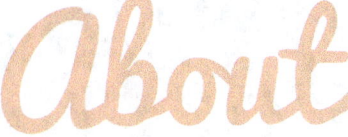

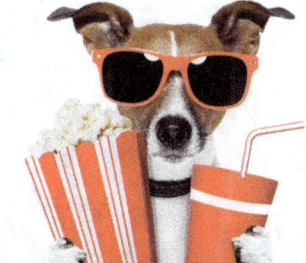

AROUND THE *House*

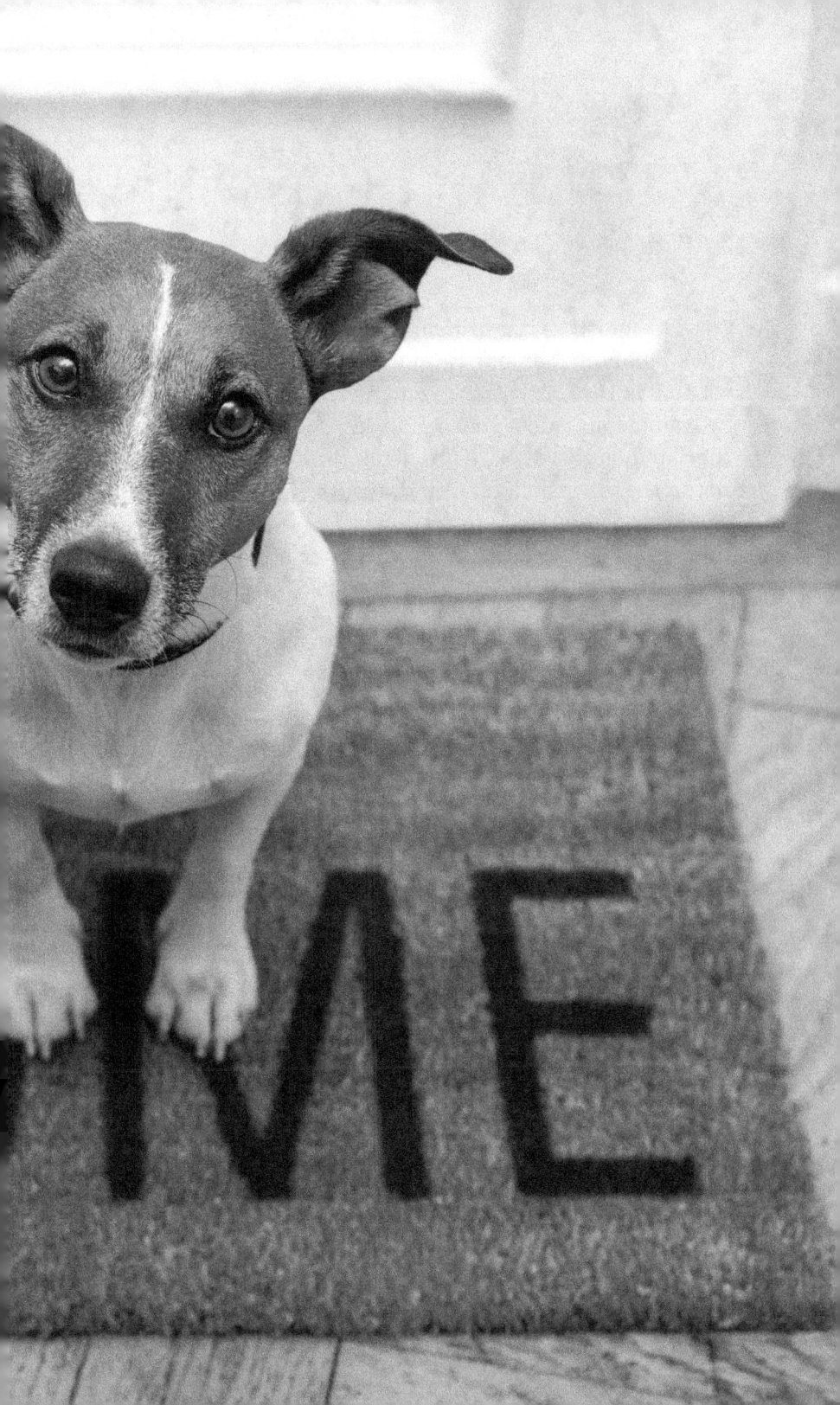

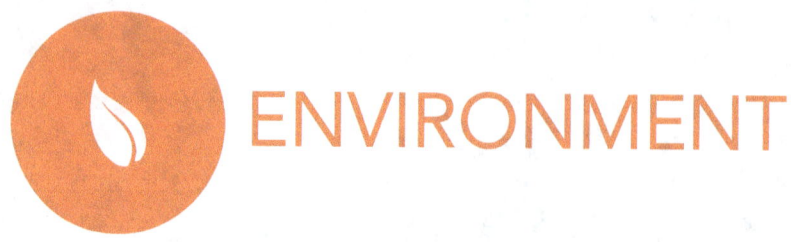

ENVIRONMENT

The most common communication breakdowns happen between family members in their own home. The good news is that this is the easiest environment to manipulate. It may not always be convenient, but it is easy. Don't try to compete with other sounds. If you want to have a meaningful conversation, turn off the television, turn off the radio, turn off the dishwasher, and turn off the washing machine. Do you want to nurture a relationship with your TV or with your spouse? It is entirely possible (and easy) to get rid of the background noise in your own home when effective communication is a priority. This is the responsibility of both communication partners.

SPEAKER

The most common speaker error in the home is talking from another room. This generally does not work, even for people with normal hearing. Your listener has hearing loss, which means it is imperative that you are face-to-face before you start speaking. A large part of your message is being received through visual cues, so they must see your face when you speak.

> Visual cues are essential for effective communication exchanges. They include body posture, facial expressions, hand gestures, and lip movements.

Listeners cannot see these important cues from another room. Your job is to go to your listener or to (nicely) request that he or she comes to you...before you begin talking. If your listener does not understand what you have said, rephrase what you said rather than repeating the same words over again. This gives your listener more information to better understand your message.

 ## LISTENER

If you want to nurture your relationship with the people you live with, you must make an effort to actively listen to them around the house. You must MAKE THEIR MESSAGE A PRIORITY, and minimize the "selective hearing loss" that so many patients admit to suffering from. If your spouse begins speaking to you while you are watching TV, then grab the remote and mute the volume for a moment. If you are in another room and hear your spouse talking to you, then go to that room, or (nicely) request that he or she comes to you. You are equally responsible for making sure you can see the speaker's face.

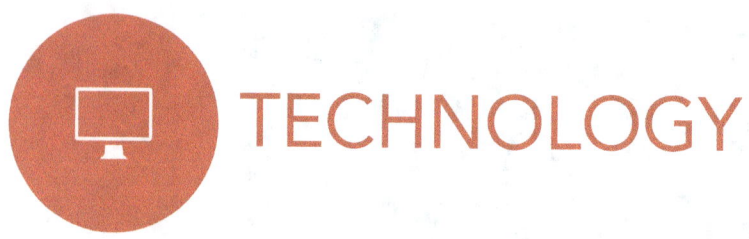

TECHNOLOGY

If you have hearing aids, wear them around the house. So often patients will take their hearing aids out when they get home to "give their ears a rest." While this is OK when you are first getting used to new hearing aids, it is absolutely unacceptable after that. People who do this are essentially saying that their "away-from-home" relationships are more important than their "in-home" relationships. WEAR YOUR HEARING AIDS AT HOME.

If watching TV is a challenge in your home, there are several great technology options. People without hearing aids can find relatively inexpensive wireless devices that send the TV signal directly from the TV to a receiver unit with headphones attached. People with hearing aids can use these devices with a neckloop and the telecoil program in their hearing aids (see "On the Phone...Technology" for more details).

The new wireless hearing aids have special accessories that deliver clear TV or stereo sound directly into the hearing aids. They also have companion microphones that can be worn by the speaker to make his or her voice loud and clear to the listener with hearing aids, even in background noise or at a distance. Be sure to ask your hearing care provider about these amazing wireless options.

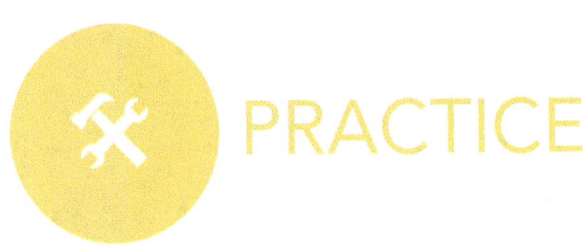

PRACTICE

Most people have spent many years developing bad communication habits around the home. They've gotten used to talking over the TV and trying to have conversations while washing the dishes. Practice and repetition of the environmental, speaker, listener, and technology tips presented here are essential to creating new habits. Experts say it takes 30 days to create a new habit. This means that for 30 days, you must be very conscious of reducing the background noise and facing each other when you talk. It may seem tedious and troublesome at first, but STICK WITH IT! Your efforts will pay off in reduced frustration and improved relationships.

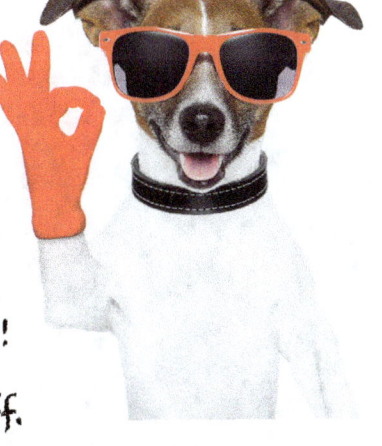

It may seem tedious and troublesome at first, but STICK WITH IT!

Your efforts will pay off.

Notes

SUCCESSFUL COMMUNICATION PLAN

Challenging Situation:

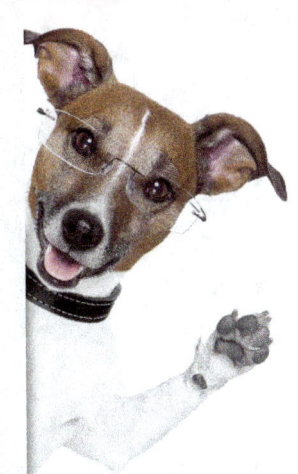

Communication Partners Involved:

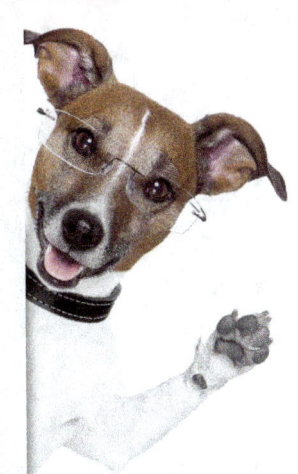 ENVIRONMENT

SPEAKER

LISTENER

TECHNOLOGY

PRACTICE

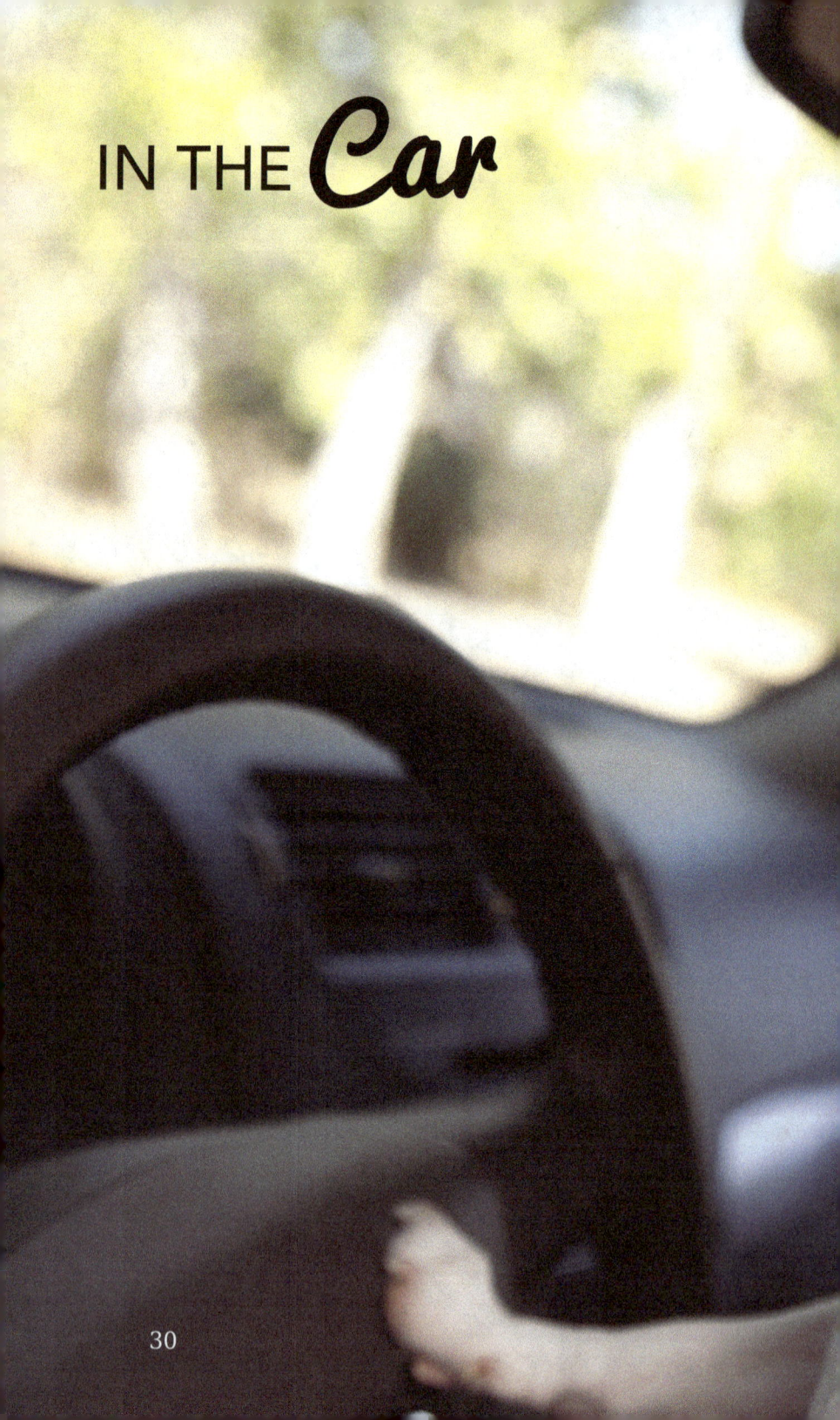

IN THE *Car*

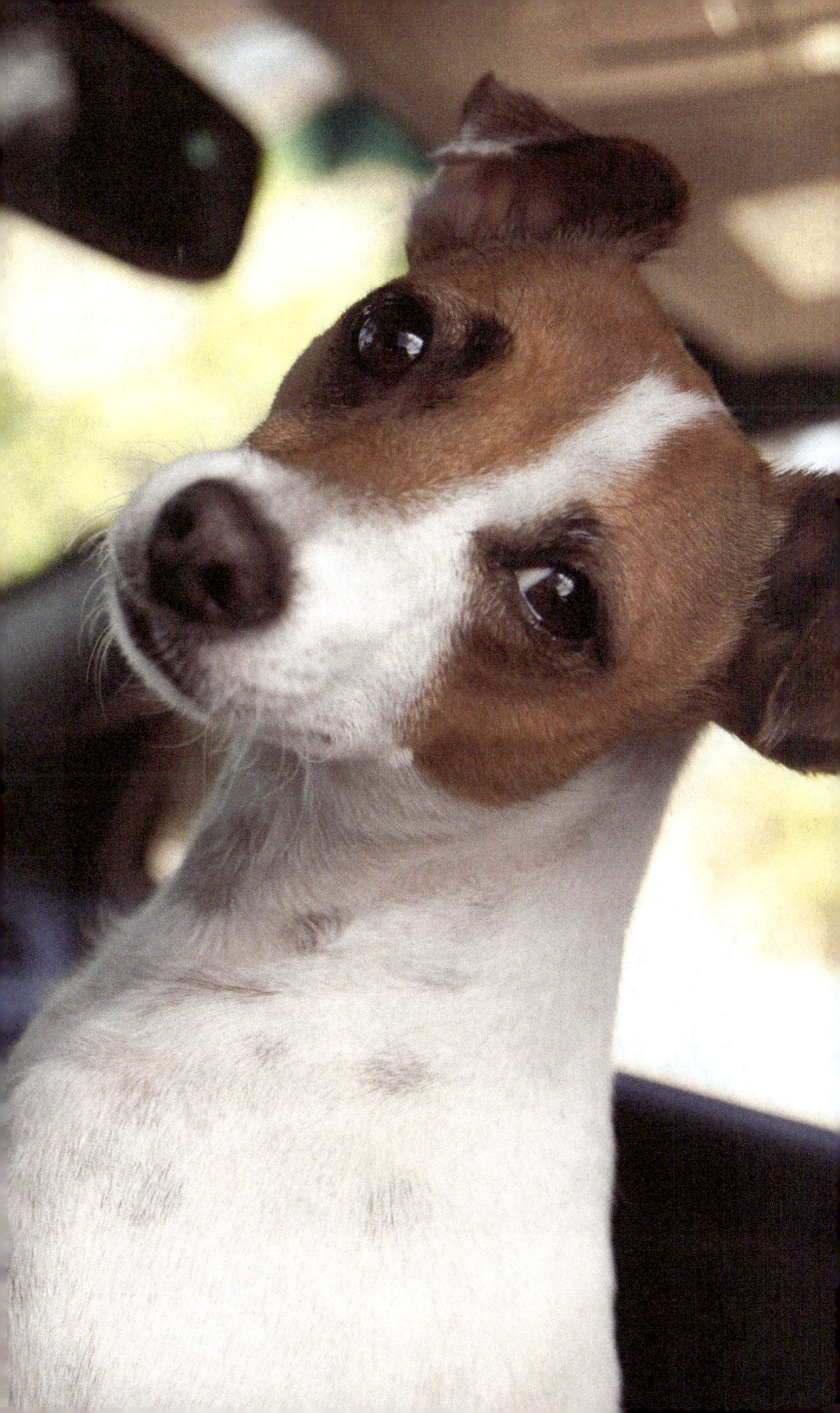

ENVIRONMENT

This is an easy environment to modify for more effective communication. Common sense tells us to first TURN OFF THE RADIO, or at least turn it down significantly when you are trying to have a conversation on the road. Similarly, make sure the car windows are closed and fans are turned off. If you have a choice of vehicles, choose the quieter car over the noisy truck when you drive together.

Road noise can be very distracting as most tires create multiple sounds that drown out conversation. However, discontinuous patterned tires create much less road noise, so ask about those for your next set of tires.

If there are more than two passengers, make sure the person with hearing loss takes the front seat. This way they can turn their body and head to hear both the driver and backseat passengers.

SPEAKER

If you are the driver, you obviously can't turn and look directly at your passenger because you need to keep your eyes on the road. But you can raise the volume of your voice a bit and enunciate clearly. And you can angle your face slightly toward your passenger rather than toward your driver's side window. Your listener must see your face. As mentioned previously, if your listener does not understand what you have said, REPHRASE what you said rather than repeating the same words over again (be ready to read this same advice for every situation).

LISTENER

If you are the driver, take control and minimize all other noises in the car. Don't be afraid to let your passengers know that you have hearing loss which makes it difficult to hear over the road noise, so you'd appreciate them speaking a bit louder in the car. If you are the passenger, which is the preferable choice in this situation, be assertive and take the passenger seat rather than the backseat. You must face your speaker to effectively receive the message over the road noise.

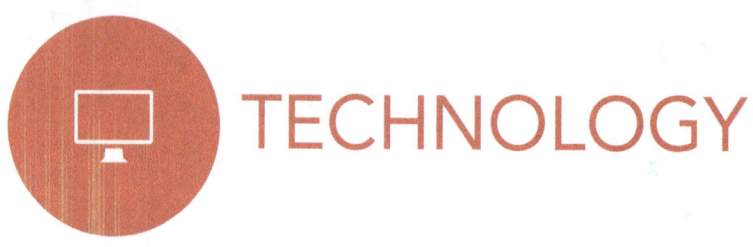

TECHNOLOGY

Most hearing aids have a special program to reduce background noise. The car is a great place to use this program. Your hearing care provider can even customize a "car" program specifically for your situation. If you are always the driver, then your "car" program can decrease the volume from your left hearing aid (so you get less road and window noise) and increase the volume on your right hearing aid (to hear your passenger better). Your provider can also maximize special noise reduction features for your "car" program that will help dramatically. But it is your responsibility to communicate this need to your hearing care provider.

If you have hearing aids with wireless capabilities, a companion microphone can be a lifesaver in the car. The speaker simply clips a small wireless microphone to his shirt which transmits his voice directly into the listener's hearing aids. There are also inexpensive wired versions of this for people who don't wear hearing aids. Ask your hearing care provider for details.

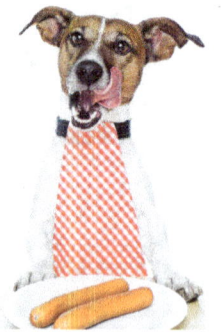

Examples of
Manual Hearing Aid Programs

- Restaurant
- Telephone
- Car
- Outdoors

- Place of Worship
- Music
- Television

Ask your hearing care provider which programs might be a good fit for you.

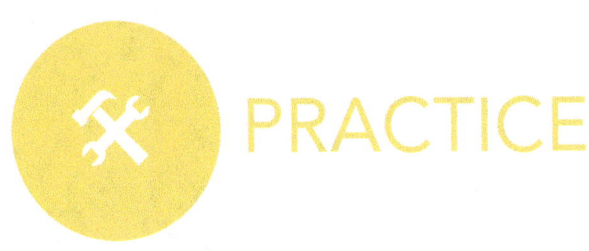

PRACTICE

The car is an easy place to practice these communication strategies. Grab a neighbor and take "practice rides" to nowhere in particular. This helps you get used to the new seating arrangement and gives you practice using the speaker and listener strategies discussed. Practice rides are also essential for adapting to new hearing aids and getting comfortable with the wireless accessories. Your hearing care provider can make adjustments to your "car" program as well as the wireless settings to make them work the best for you. However, this can only be accomplished after you have practiced with them so that you can give your provider clear feedback about what needs to be adjusted.

"I wish I had received a copy of this book from my audiologist when I got my first pair of hearing aids eight years ago. It would have made such a difference as I adapted to life with hearing aids."
— SARAH, SPEAK-UP LIBRARIAN BLOGGER

Notes

SUCCESSFUL COMMUNICATION PLAN

Challenging Situation:

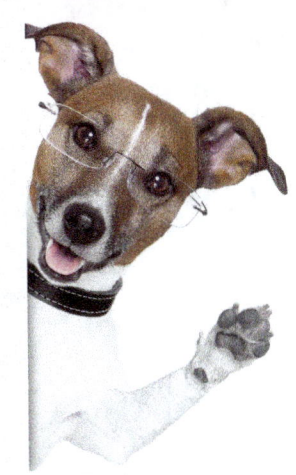

Communication Partners Involved:

⬤ ENVIRONMENT

⬤ SPEAKER

⬤ LISTENER

⬤ TECHNOLOGY

⬤ PRACTICE

Download blank communication plans at www.5keys.info

DINING *Out*

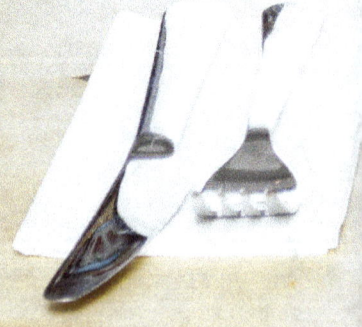

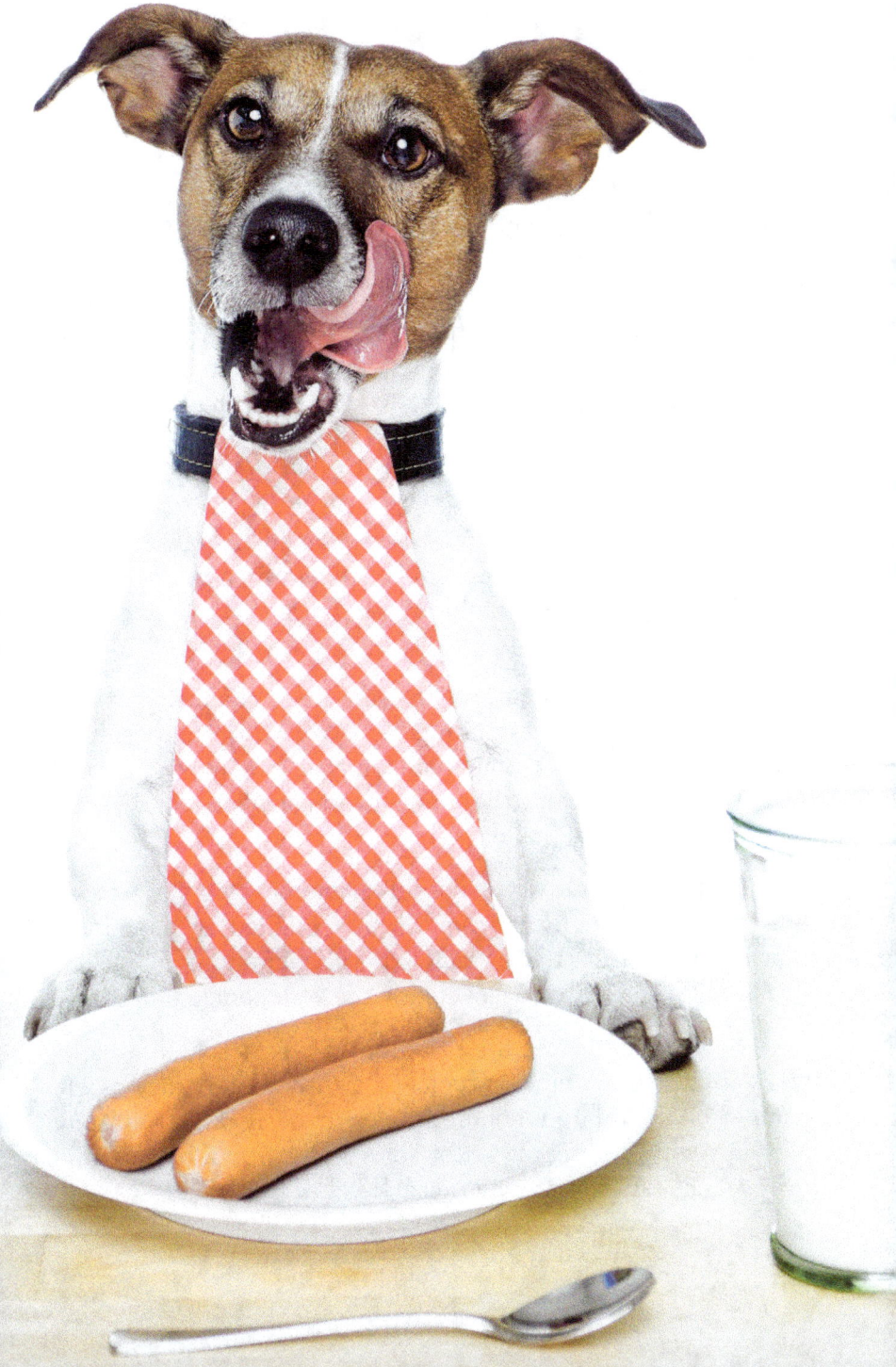

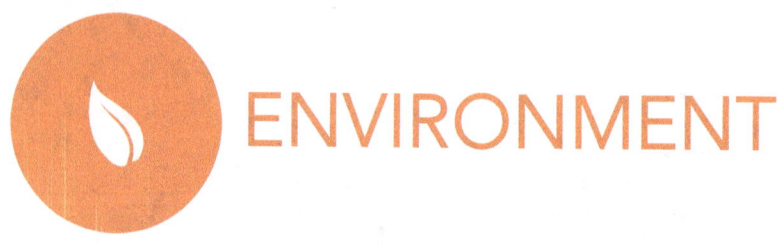

ENVIRONMENT

Noisy restaurants may be the most difficult listening situation for people with hearing loss. The problem is that restaurant noise tends to be a lower pitch, and most hearing losses tend to be in the higher pitches. This leaves the hearing impaired person with very little to work with in terms of sound input. It is also a bit more challenging to modify a restaurant environment than it is to make environmental changes in your car or home. But don't worry! There are several strategies that work very well. You just need to be assertive and know that YOU ARE IN CONTROL OF WHERE AND WHEN YOU EAT. Be very open and honest with your friends and family members so that they are aware of your hearing challenges when you go out to eat. Make suggestions to help plan an outing that will be more fun for everyone.

First, choose restaurants that are more conducive to conversation. These are restaurants that have a quiet ambiance, without music blaring through hidden speakers in every corner. Also, choose restaurants that have several smaller rooms rather than one huge dining hall.

Request a booth or corner table, and be willing to wait an extra few minutes for that request to be fulfilled. Select a table that is farther from the entrance or kitchen, and one that has good lighting so that you can clearly see your companion's face.

Second, go to restaurants during off-peak hours, especially if you are going to a typically crowded and noisy establishment. Plan a late lunch at 2pm or an early dinner at 4pm. Not only will you receive faster service, but you'll be listening over much less background noise.

SPEAKER

Going out to eat is a treat that should be enjoyed by all parties, and it is your responsibility to make sure your hearing-impaired dining partner is part of this enjoyment. Be flexible with the choice of restaurant, dining time, and seating choice. Help to seat the person with hearing loss at the quietest part of the table. If your listener has a better ear, give her the part of the table where that better ear has the advantage.

If you are dining with a group of three or more people, know that it is very difficult for someone with hearing loss to follow multiple conversations. Make an effort to keep side conversations to a minimum and check-in frequently to see if any clarification is needed. For example, "Nancy, were you able to hear Dan's joke?"

Discuss the menu ahead of time so that you can provide any clarification needed when it is time to order. Get your listener's attention before you start speaking by calling her name or tapping her shoulder. Remember to speak slowly, distinctly, and directly to your listener.

Choose restaurants that have several smaller rooms rather than one huge dining hall. Plan ahead and make reservations for the restaurant and table that you prefer.

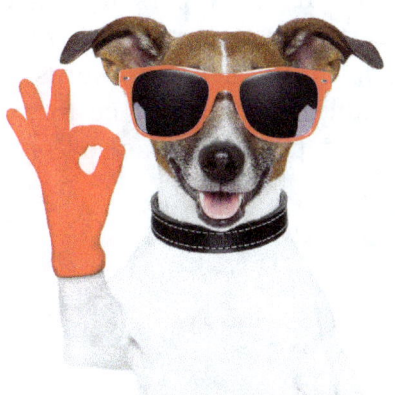

It is OK to speak slightly louder, but do not shout or exaggerate your words.

If your listener misses part of the conversation, rephrase what was said rather than repeating the same words over again.

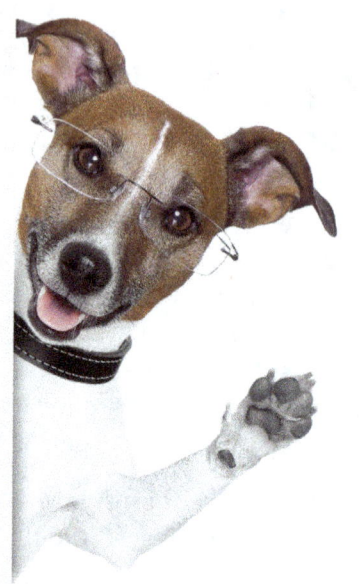

Position yourself so the listener can clearly see your face. Make sure there is good lighting but that the light is not shining directly in the eyes of your listener. Avoid talking with food in your mouth, or with your hands, napkins, or other objects in front of your mouth. Try not to turn your head away from the person while speaking. If your listener misses part of the conversation, rephrase what was said rather than repeating the same words over again. Finally, try to avoid sudden changes in the topic of conversation without clearly alerting your listener to the change.

LISTENER

You are ultimately in control of where and when you dine out, so choose wisely. Noisy restaurants are where "active listening" really comes into play. This means being fully present in the moment so that you are aware of the surroundings that might become a topic of conversation. For example, become familiar with the menu and read the specials ahead of time.

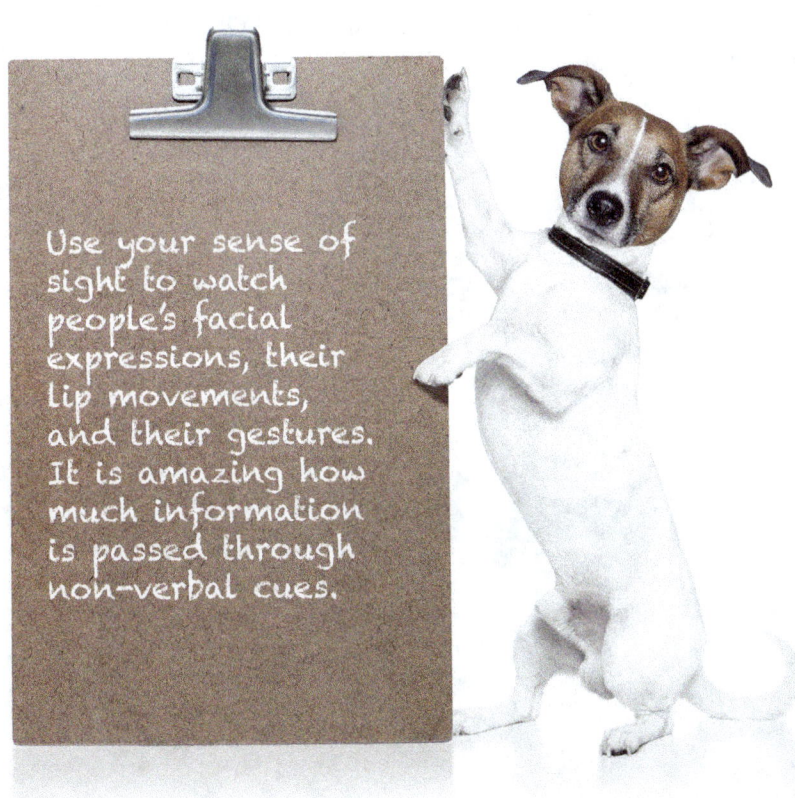

Use your sense of sight to watch people's facial expressions, their lip movements, and their gestures. It is amazing how much information is passed through non-verbal cues.

If you are dining with a group, concentrate on one conversation at a time. It is difficult for people with normal hearing to follow multiple conversations, so don't expect to be able to do this with hearing loss. Be sure to sit next to the person that you most want to converse with and enjoy your conversation with that person. He or she will probably be the person who is most likely to provide you with clarification about the other conversations.

Finally, part of "active listening" means actively tuning out the noises that aren't helpful for communication. This can be particularly tough when you first get hearing aids, but it gets easier with practice. Of course you will hear silverware clanking, dishes banging, babies crying, and people laughing. These are all normal sounds of a noisy restaurant. Your job is to learn to actively tune out those sounds and PUT YOUR FULL FOCUS ON THE CONVERSATION AT YOUR TABLE. This listening technique will be a huge help to you in many difficult listening situations, so practice it every chance you get!

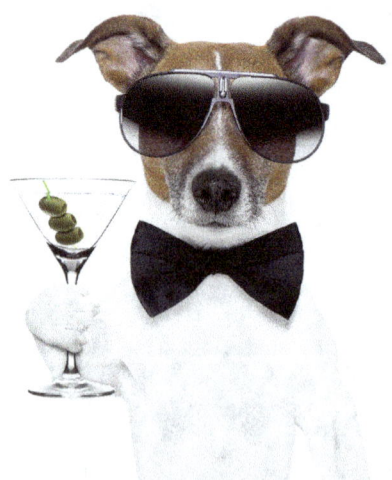

Your job is to learn to actively tune out background noise and put your full focus on the conversation at your table.

TECHNOLOGY

If you wear hearing aids, it is imperative that you wear them in restaurants. This will be the most difficult environment for you to adapt to using hearing aids. The hearing aids (even the really expensive hearing aids) do not know that their owner wants to hear the conversation to their front-left rather than the louder conversation that happens to be taking place to their front-right. Some people talk louder than others, and today's hearing aids are made to pick up speech. If someone at a neighboring table has a louder voice, the hearing aids will naturally pick up on that rather than your soft-spoken dining companion. Therefore, it is up to YOU to CHOOSE to focus on the voice of your companion rather than the voices coming from the other tables. This takes time and practice, but will only get easier if you wear your hearing aids every time you go to a restaurant.

Most hearing aids will have a "restaurant" program that can be accessed by pressing a button on the hearing aids or on a remote control unit. This special program will help to tune out noises behind you, and may soften some of the clanking noises that can be irritating in a restaurant.

Again, for those who have wireless technology in their hearing aids, the companion microphone can be a dinner-saver when dining with one other person. The speaker simply attaches the microphone to a shirt collar, and the listener's hearing aids can be tuned in only to that speaker, thus eliminating all of the other restaurant noise. This is a wonderful communication tool, but can become irritating if the speaker is a noisy eater! When dining with a group, the wireless microphone can be placed at the far-end of the table to make it easier for the listener to hear speakers who are farther away.

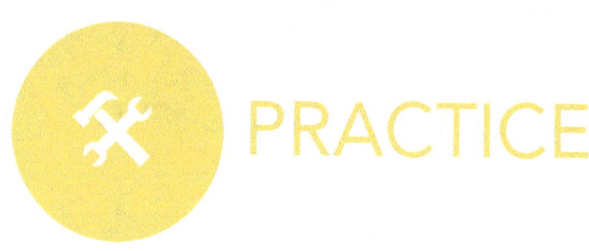

PRACTICE

If you keep going back to the same noisy restaurant, then chances are you'll have the same communication frustrations. Experiment with different restaurants. When you find one that you really like, experiment with different tables to find the area with the least amount of background noise. Next, experiment with each seat at that table to determine where you hear the best. Each of these "experimental dining experiences" is an opportunity for both the speaker and the listener to practice the strategies discussed.

Don't give up after one noisy meal. Each dining experience will get easier. This practice will also help you to give your hearing care provider accurate feedback about your experience so that he or she can make the adjustments needed for optimal hearing in this situation. Dining out will once again be a pleasant experience!

> It is critical for those with hearing aids to practice using the hearing aids and the wireless accessories in this challenging environment. Now you have an excellent excuse to try a new restaurant every week!

SUCCESSFUL COMMUNICATION PLAN

Challenging Situation:

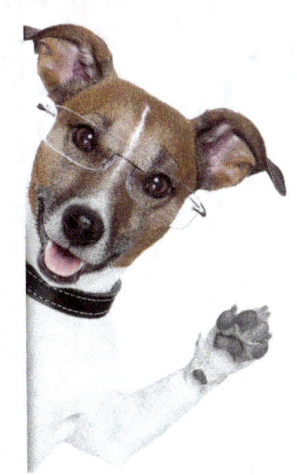

Communication Partners Involved:

ENVIRONMENT

SPEAKER

LISTENER

TECHNOLOGY

PRACTICE

ON THE *Phone*

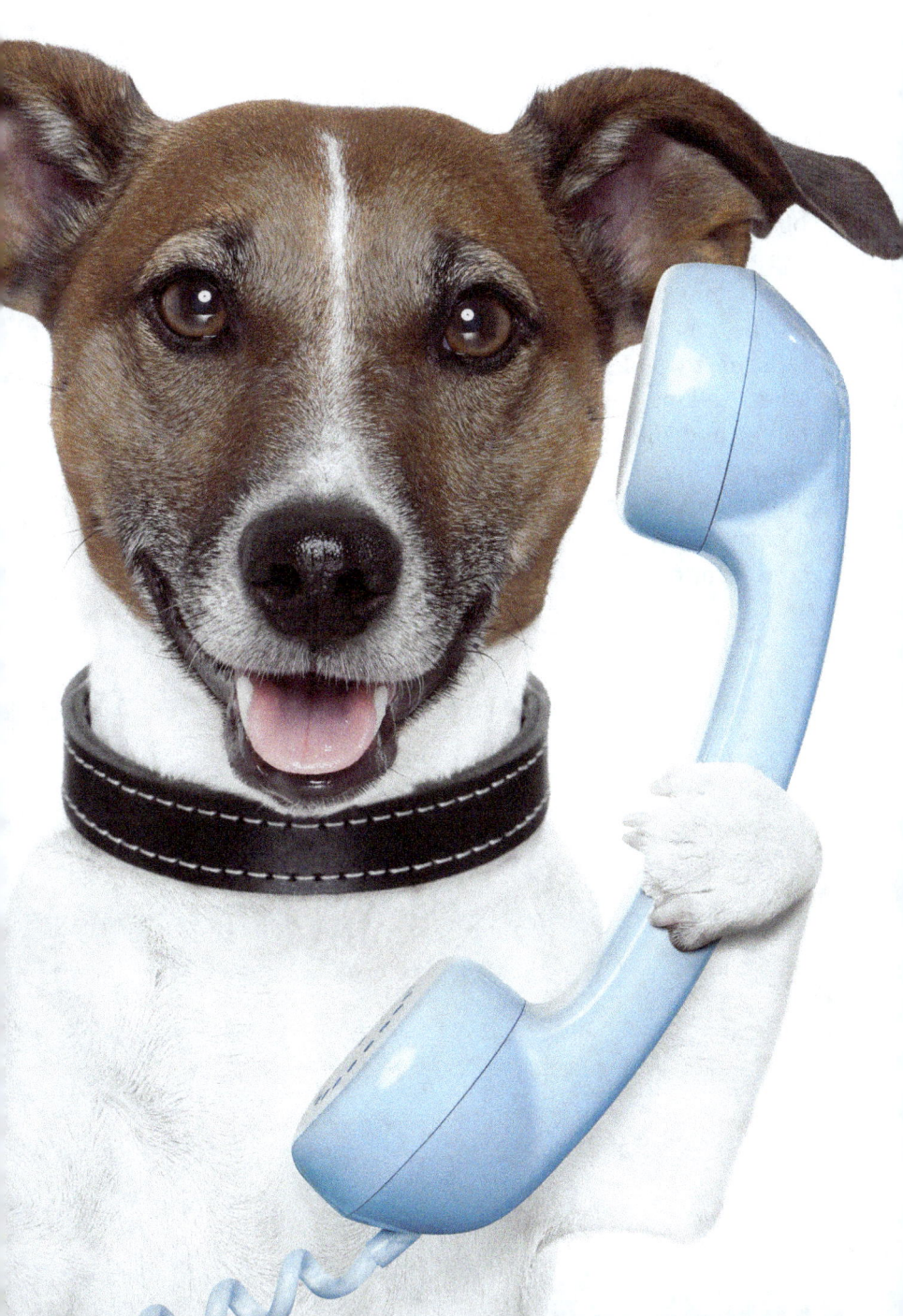

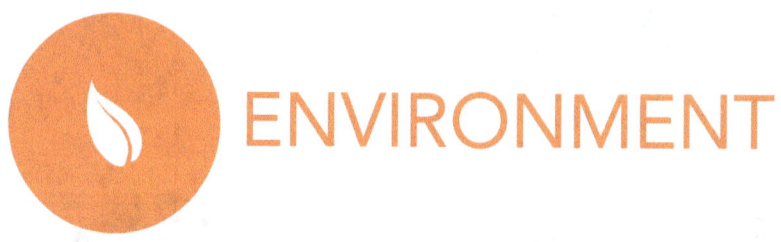

ENVIRONMENT

There are two main reasons why telephone conversations can present a communication challenge. First, the listener obviously cannot see the speaker's face, therefore visual cues are not possible. Second, the clarity of the speaker's voice is dependent upon the clarity of the phone they are using as well as the connection between the two phones. Common sense tells us to make sure all background noise is turned down when talking on the phone. This means turning off the TV, radio, and dishwasher. Landline telephones typically have a cleaner signal than cellular phones, so choose the landline phone at home or at work if there is an option. If you work in a noisy environment, walk into an unused room to conduct the conversation.

Our family now has all the tools we need to help deal with my hearing loss because, as we are finding, the frustrations are real."
— RITA C.

SPEAKER

Use a landline phone if possible. If using a cellular phone, do not use a wireless or hands-free device because your voice will not come through as clearly. Hold the phone close to your mouth and avoid doing other things while you speak so that you aren't moving the phone around. Speak slowly and enunciate clearly, but do not exaggerate your words.

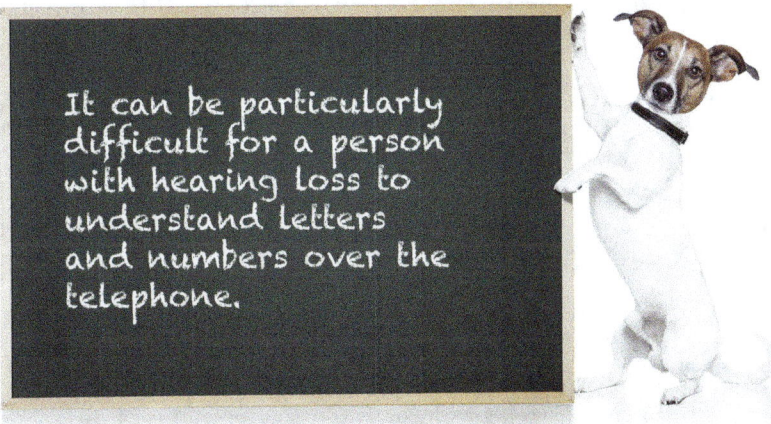

It can be particularly difficult for a person with hearing loss to understand letters and numbers over the telephone.

If you are saying an address, phone number, or other piece of information that contains letters and numbers, it is important to give additional clues. For example, "C as in Charlie" or "P as in Paul." The numbers "nine" and "five" are especially difficult to distinguish over the phone, so provide clarification such as, "Nine, as in the number before ten." As with every other situation, REPHRASE rather than repeat the sentence or word that was missed.

LISTENER

Use the telephone you feel has the best sound quality and turn the volume up to a comfortable level. Some listeners prefer to use their speakerphone so they can hear the speaker with both of their ears rather than just one. If you miss something the speaker has said, ask them to REPHRASE their last sentence.

If the speaker is giving you numbers or letters, ask YES or NO questions to clarify what was said. This is a good clarification strategy in any environment, but especially so on the telephone when you cannot see the speaker's lips. For example, let's say your speaker tells you to meet them at five. But you aren't sure if they said five or nine so you ask them, "Did you say five or nine?" By asking the question this way, the speaker will simply say the same word over again, and chances are you will miss it the second and third time they say that difficult word. Now let's clarify with our YES/NO strategy and ask them, "Did you say nine?" Given that this is a YES/NO question, your speaker will say, "No" (which is a nice and easy word to hear over the telephone, even for people with hearing loss), "I said five." This way, your clarification has taken place with one simple question.

Another great strategy is to repeat back what you THINK you heard. This lets your speaker know exactly where the communication breakdown has occurred, so he or she can clarify the incorrect part rather than having to repeat the entire sentence over again. It also shows that you are indeed listening attentively.

The word "what?" often implies that you weren't paying attention, or were distracted by something else in your environment. It is truly the LAZY way of asking for clarification.

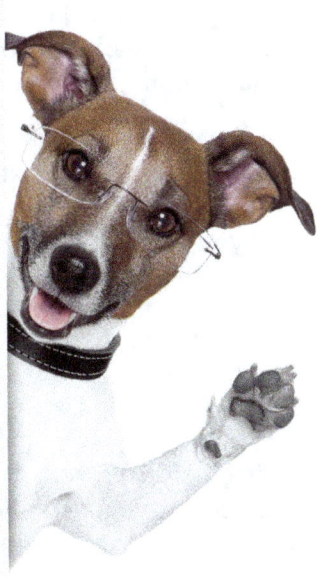

"This handbook has helped me understand what I can and cannot expect from my hearing aids."
— SYLVIA A.

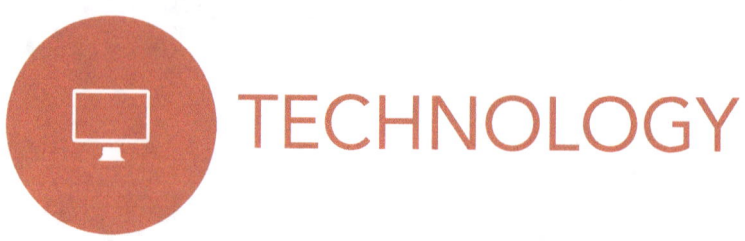

TECHNOLOGY

There are so many options when it comes to technological help with the telephone, that there really is no excuse for telephone communication breakdowns.

We'll start by discussing technology for people who do not have hearing aids. First, if you are struggling to hear on the telephone, there is a good chance that you need hearing aids, and you really should explore this option. The technology that is available for people with hearing aids is amazing.

If you haven't made that investment in yourself yet, you need to start with a good telephone. There are landline and mobile phones that have volume controls and extra loud speakers. These will help to some extent, and are good for people with hearing aids as well. If you are purchasing a new mobile phone, be sure to choose one that is "hearing aid compatible" with a microphone (M) and telecoil (T) rating of 3 or 4.

There are special phones and services that provide a typewritten version of the verbal message that is coming through. These are called TTY (TeleTypewriter) or TDD (Telecommunication Device for the Deaf). There are also special relay services if the person making the call doesn't have a TTY. Captioned telephones offer users the ability to amplify conversations while viewing the captions on a large display screen. Several companies provide captioned phones and the captioning service free of charge, as well as free in-home installation and training. Ask your hearing care provider about the services available in your area, and see the Resources at the end of this handbook.

The text messaging capabilities on mobile phones can be very helpful for sending a quick message, especially one that includes details with numbers and letters. There are also TTY adapters for newer cell phones. Most phones have a headphone

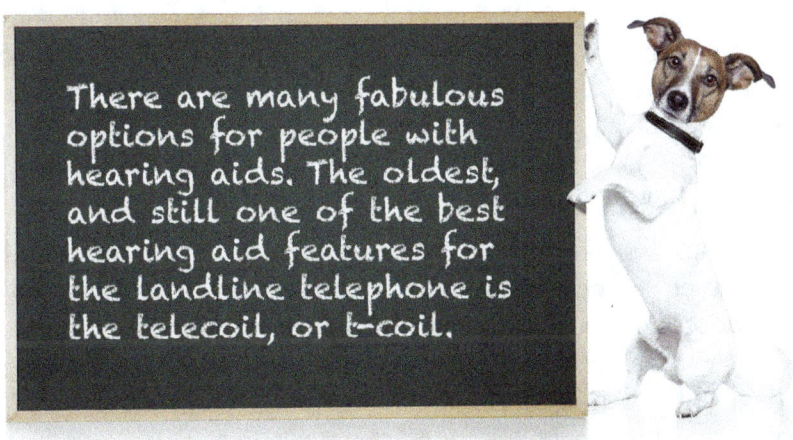

There are many fabulous options for people with hearing aids. The oldest, and still one of the best hearing aid features for the landline telephone is the telecoil, or t-coil.

jack in which you can plug a high quality pair of headphones so that you hear the speaker in both ears. Just remember that you still must hold your phone's microphone up to your mouth when you speak.

Video messaging is a fantastic alternative to telephone use, and is available on most computers, tablets, and smart phones. Video messaging enables listeners to see the speaker's face so they can read the lip movements and other facial expressions that provide so much valuable information.

The telecoil is a small metal coil inside the hearing aid that picks up electromagnetic energy, which a landline telephone naturally emits. Most hearing aids come standard with t-coils, but it is a good idea to make sure that yours will come with them if you are purchasing a new pair. If you aren't sure if your hearing aids have a t-coil, just ask your hearing care provider. The beauty of the t-coil is that it works independently of your microphone, so it only picks up sound from the telephone. This naturally blocks out all other surrounding sounds, making it easier to hear the speaker.

The newer wireless hearing aids provide the amazing ability to hear your phone conversation directly in your hearing aids. This happens with different streaming devices that pick up the sound from your phone and send it directly into your hearing aids. You simply wear a device around your neck or have it sitting near you (different manufacturers' devices work differently), and have a clear conversation without ever touching your telephone. Some smart phones work directly with the hearing aids so that a streaming device is not needed. Your hearing care provider can give you more details about this exciting new option.

Wireless hearing aid devices work with mobile phones that are equipped with Bluetooth™ technology. There are simple adaptations that can make this work with landline phones as well, but a separate cord is usually needed. Many hearing aids also have a "binaural phone" feature. This works for both home and mobile phones without any additional cords. The hearing aid user simply holds the phone up to one ear, and the hearing aid on that side sends the sound to the other hearing aid so that a clear telephone signal is coming into both ears.

The telecommunication technology available for people with hearing loss is changing so quickly that this description may be a bit outdated by the time you read this! Just be sure to ask your hearing care provider about your options and know that the technology is available to enable clear communication on the telephone.

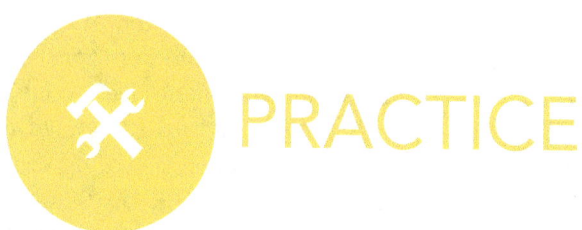 PRACTICE

Bad telephone habits are sometimes hard to break, but practice can make perfect. Experiment with different telephones. Try the speakerphone or headphones. If you wear hearing aids, practice with your t-coil or wireless technology. These may seem awkward at first, but with practice you will come to appreciate the amazing clarity that this new technology can provide.

SUCCESSFUL COMMUNICATION PLAN

Challenging Situation:

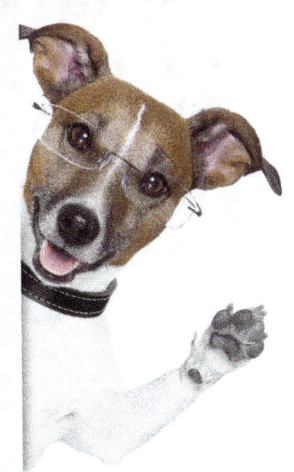

Communication Partners Involved:

⬤ ENVIRONMENT

⬤ SPEAKER

⬤ LISTENER

⬤ TECHNOLOGY

⬤ PRACTICE

PUBLIC *Events*

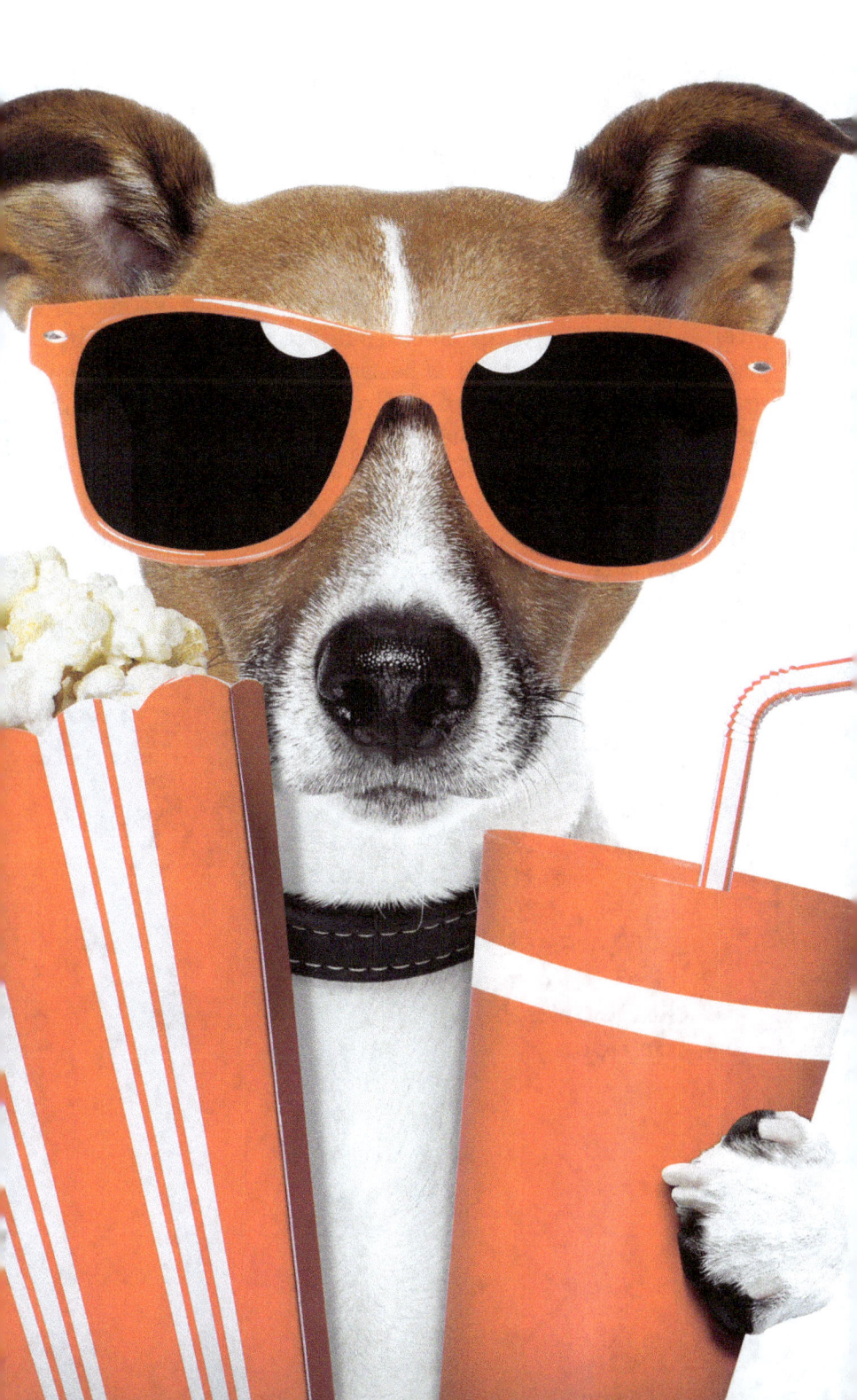

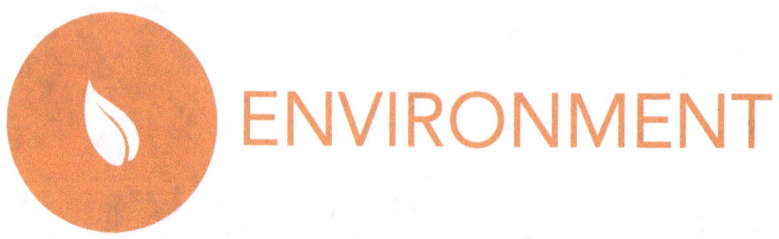

ENVIRONMENT

The main environmental modification you have control over is WHERE YOU SIT. You should experiment to find the seating location that has the best acoustics for you. This will probably be near the middle or front of the room, but it can depend greatly on the venue. Once you find the best "acoustic" seat for you, make sure to plan ahead, purchase your tickets early, and be willing to pay a bit more. Sometimes the more expensive tickets give you the best seating options. If concerts, plays, and musicals are an important part of your life, then you owe yourself this luxury.

If the seating is open, as it usually is in churches or large meetings, plan to ARRIVE EXTRA EARLY to get the seat that works best for you.

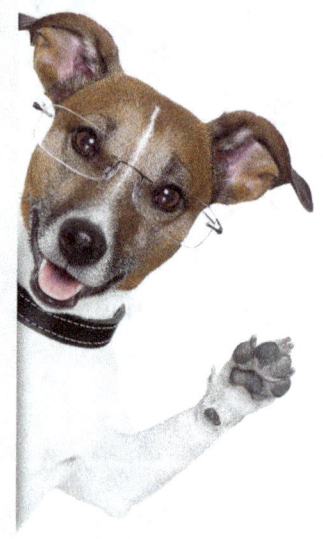

SPEAKER

The speakers in this situation will be the performers, or the people leading the event or meeting. Obviously performers may be limited in their ability to modify their speech, depending on the nature of the performance. If you are an event speaker or leader, it is your responsibility to ensure your message is coming through loud and clear.

Always test the microphone prior to starting, and use a lapel microphone if you will be moving around. Avoid gesturing if you are using a handheld microphone, as the resulting fluctuations in volume can make it very difficult to hear.

Speak slowly, enunciate clearly, and frequently check in with your audience for signs of comprehension and interest. A simple question such as, "Am I coming through loud and clear?" will pull attention to you.

Watch for signs of active listening such as heads nodding in agreement, smiles, or laughs. Also watch for signs that your message may not be coming through clearly, such as glazed eyes or a drooping head.

Your message may be fabulous, but a message that is difficult to hear will always be boring to those who aren't receiving it clearly.

LISTENER

If you are attending a performance or event, become familiar with the theme and flow of the event beforehand. Watch a recorded version, read the handbook, watch the movie, or listen to the audio. Before the event starts, read the entire program. If you have an idea of what to expect next, you will be able to follow and thus enjoy the performance.

Public events should not be difficult listening situations for you if you plan ahead and sit where you can see and hear the best. You must be able to see the speaker's face, which means you must sit close to the front. Watch facial expressions as well as lip movements.

Plan ahead so you'll know what the event is about. Read the program or agenda before it starts, and anticipate the topics of conversation. Know that it is perfectly normal to miss a word or two here and there. Don't give up and blame your hearing loss! Chances are that others missed the word as well, and you'll be able to catch it the next time around. Continue to listen, and keep your eyes on the speaker.

Meetings in the workplace or the community can be very challenging for those with hearing loss. Competing sounds such as side conversations, the clicking of multiple people typing at once, traffic noise, and heating or air conditioning fans can be very distracting. As the listener, it is your responsibility to seat yourself in the middle of the group and look directly at the speaker. Ask for an agenda beforehand to help you follow the topics, and ask for a final summary at the conclusion. Be attentive and do not multi-task or do other work as you may lose the flow of the discourse.

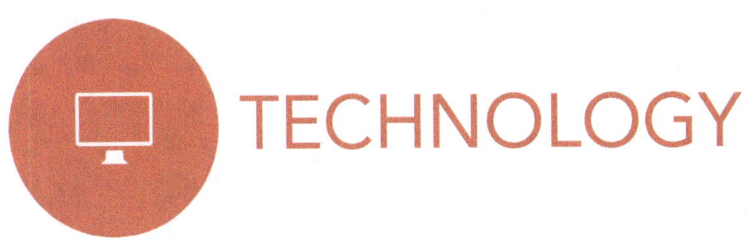

TECHNOLOGY

Many public establishments are required by law to have technological assistance for people with hearing loss. You will find this information on their website, or by calling the venue. There are often special headphones that you can check out at the ticket office or lobby. These are typically used without hearing aids. You need to plan ahead and arrive early to use these assistive listening devices. Unfortunately, the venues sometimes do not have enough to accommodate all of the people who need them. They may also not be diligent about making sure the batteries are good, so be sure to test yours before taking your seat.

For those with hearing aids, there are several great options. First, you may have a special program in your hearing aids for this type of event. For example, your hearing care provider can create a special program that is tailored to large rooms. Second, you have the option of using the venue's assistive listening devices. Public venues are required to provide headphones for those who do not wear hearing aids and to provide neckloops for people who do wear hearing aids. When using a neckloop, you simply put your hearing aids in the t-coil program. If your hearing aids don't have t-coils (ask your provider to be sure) you may use the venue's headphones or ask your provider about wireless devices that are equipped with t-coils and connect to your hearing aids via Bluetooth technology.

Arguably the best option for people with hearing aids is to choose a venue that is equipped with a hearing loop. Large area induction loops are becoming more common in public venues, which is exciting considering their incredible benefit to people with hearing loss. People with hearing aids simply switch their hearing aids to the t-coil setting, and the sound is delivered directly into their hearing aids! People without hearing aids can check out receivers and headphones to use with the loop system as well. For more information about induction loops, and to check for them in your area, go to www.hearingloop.org.

Those with wireless capabilities in their hearing aids may also be able to use remote microphones at certain public events. This works especially well for meetings or lectures where there is one speaker who is relatively close to you (most wireless microphones transmit up to 30 feet). The speaker simply wears the companion microphone, and his or her voice is delivered straight to your hearing aids. Be sure to ask your hearing care provider about this option.

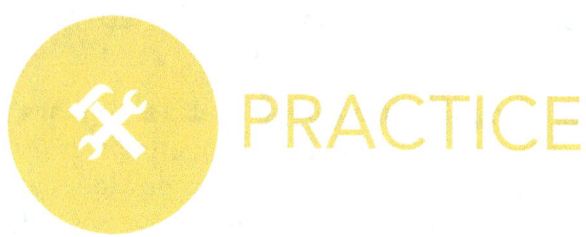

PRACTICE

Here is yet another excuse to get out there and enjoy the beautiful sounds of life! Public venues are great places to practice what you have learned here. Many are free, and the seating is often open so you can try different seating options to determine where you hear and see the best.

You may need to do some re-search to find the public venues that have special accommodations for people with hearing loss. You should become familiar with this symbol, which is your clue that the venue is equipped with technology to help people with hearing loss.

If the venue is equipped with a large area loop system, you'll see a similar symbol, but with a "T" in the lower right corner.

For people with hearing aids, practice with your different hearing aid programs and accessories is crucial to your success. The more you practice, the better feedback you can provide to your hearing care providers so they can make the necessary adjustments.

The modern hearing aids and their wireless accessories can drastically improve hearing in these public venues. However, regular and timely follow up appointments with your hearing care professional are critical for the fine tuning adjustments that may be necessary for optimal hearing.

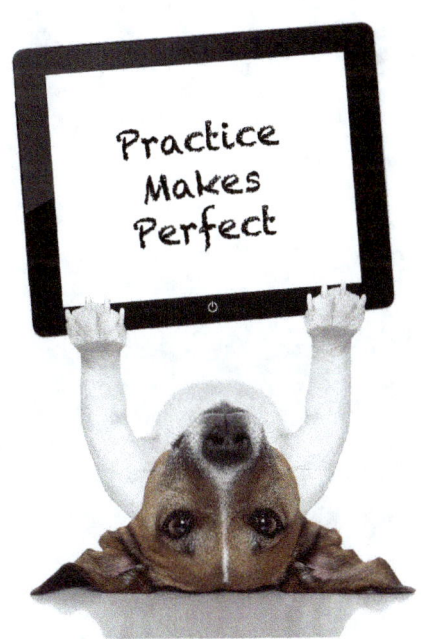

Notes

SUCCESSFUL COMMUNICATION PLAN

Challenging Situation:

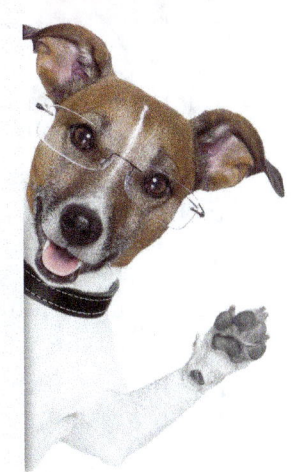

Communication Partners Involved:

● ENVIRONMENT

● SPEAKER

● LISTENER

● TECHNOLOGY

● PRACTICE

Download blank communication plans at www.5keys.info

FINAL THOUGHTS

Yes, hearing loss can certainly present a communication challenge. However, it should not prevent you from enjoying all that life has to offer! You can significantly reduce communication breakdowns by making a few common sense modifications to your environment, implementing effective speaking and listening strategies, and investing in the amazing technology that is available today.

It should now be perfectly clear that the responsibility for improving communication does not fall solely on the shoulders of the person with hearing loss. The people who talk to that person on a regular basis are just as responsible for learning and practicing the keys discussed in this handbook.

Create a Successful Communication Plan that lists where and with whom your personal communication breakdowns most often occur. Once you've identified the most challenging situations, you can apply what you've learned in this handbook by writing out the Environmental, Speaker, Listener, Technology, and Practice strategies you'll use to ensure a successful communication exchange. Then post your plan where you'll see it every single day. Make sure all parties involved have a copy as well. You'll be amazed how much this little exercise helps to break bad habits and improve your communication. You can use the plans included in this handbook, or download blank Successful Communication Plans at www.5keys.info.

The choice is yours. Will you let hearing loss keep you from going to restaurants with your family? Will you stop talking on the phone with your mother or father because they can't hear you? Will you try to hide your hearing loss and fake your way through conversations at home and at work? Will you use your hearing loss as an excuse to withdraw from the world?

Alternatively, will you choose to take control of your hearing loss? Will you make those reservations in the quiet section of your favorite restaurant ahead of time so that you can enjoy a conversation with your family? Will you help your hearing impaired parents to hear you on the phone by speaking clearly, or even buying them a nice amplified telephone for their birthday? Will you kindly remind your coworkers, friends, and family about your hearing loss and educate them about ways to communicate more effectively with you? Will you use the strategies and technology suggestions in this handbook to jump back into the world of sound, knowing that you are empowered and prepared to tackle any difficult listening situation?

At Cut to the Chase Communication, we are confident that you will make the right choice. We believe that you want to continue to build and nurture the relationships that are most important in your life. We trust that you and your loved ones will implement and practice what you have learned in this handbook. You are now equipped with the Five Keys to Communication Success!

Yes, hearing loss can certainly present challenges, but it should not prevent you from enjoying all that life has to offer. Make the most of these Five Keys to Communication Success and enjoy every day!

ONLINE RESOURCES

Hearing Loss Organizations, Associations and Communities

American Academy of Audiology
www.HowsYourHearing.org

American Academy of Doctors of Audiology, Patient Resources
www.audiologist.org/patient/patient-resources

American Tinnitus Association
www.ata.org

Association for Late-Defeaned Adults, Inc.
www.alda.org

Better Hearing Institute
www.BetterHearing.org

Cut to the Chase Communication, LLC
www.5keys.info

Hear Well Stay Vital
www.HearWellStayVital.org

Hearing Like Me
www.HearingLikeMe.com

Hearing Loss Association of America
www.HearingLoss.org

Ida Institute
www.IdaInstitute.com

Think Audiology
www.ThinkAudiology.com

Technology Resources

ADCO Hearing Products, Inc.
www.adcoHearing.com

Assist 2 Hear, LLC
www.assist2hear.com

CapTel
www.captel.com

Caption Call
www.captioncall.com

clEAR Auditory Brain Training
www.clearworks4ears.com

Harris Communications
www.HarrisComm.com

Hearing Loops
www.HearingLoop.org

Neurotone Sound Thinking
www.neurotone.com

Sound Success Rehabilitation Resource
www.abrehabportal.com

**Telecommunications for the Deaf
and Hard of Hearing, Inc.**
www.tdiforaccess.org

ABOUT THE AUTHOR

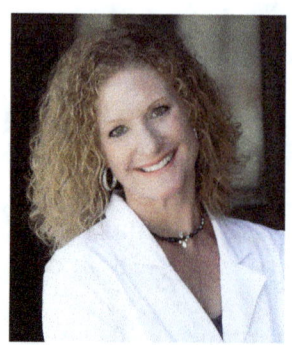

Dr. Dusty Jessen was drawn to the field of Communication Disorders after years of observing and interacting with several family members who had speech and hearing challenges. She earned her Doctorate in Audiology from the Arizona School of Health Sciences and spent 15 years as the Director of Audiology in a busy Ear, Nose, and Throat clinic. She now owns and operates a private practice audiology clinic where she specializes in adult hearing rehabilitation. Dr. Jessen is passionate about helping her patients and their family members overcome the frustrations that accompany hearing loss. She lives in Centennial, Colorado, with her husband and their two sons.

In 2013, Dr Jessen created the 5 Keys Communication counseling program to educate and empower people affected by hearing loss. Since then, she has spoken for countless consumer and professional organizations and published numerous articles about the importance of utilizing effective communication strategies. The 5 Keys Communication consumer handouts have been translated into multiple languages and the program is being used across the United States and in many countries around the world.

Dr. Jessen welcomes your questions, comments, and suggestions. Please visit her website or contact her via e-mail.

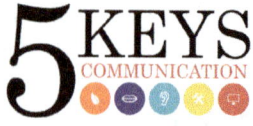

www.5keys.info

support@5keys.org

www.ingramcontent.com/pod-product-compliance
Lightning Source LLC
Chambersburg PA
CBHW062110280526
45788CB00003B/1415